PROSTATE CANCER

THE LIFE AND TIMES OF A SURVIVOR

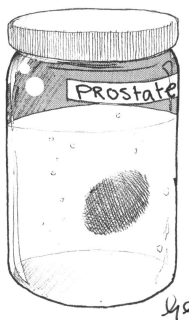

George Sayell

GEORGE SAYELL

ILLUSTRATIONS BY ANDY WATT

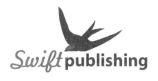

Swift publishing

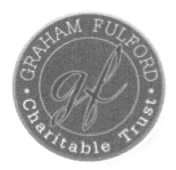

Swift Publishing Ltd,
145-157, St John Street,
London,
EC1V 4PW

First published by Swift Publishing in 2015

ISBN: 978-0-9927154-6-5

CONTENTS

FOREWORD

The writer of this saga was referred to me at the Queen Elizabeth Hospital, Birmingham, in 2007 aged 68 having been diagnosed with 'early prostate cancer'. He was assessed and found to be extremely fit, highly motivated and of a suitable age for treatment by Laparoscopic Radical Prostatectomy (keyhole surgery) to remove the organ. Following counselling the operation was carried out a few months later. The removed organ was examined and there was no sign of cancer having escaped prior to the operation.

There are a number of possible side effects with this operation, all of which are discussed with the patient during the pre-op counselling. The main ones are Incontinence, Erectile Dysfunction and consequential damage. These generally are self-correcting or are easily resolved by medication or minor surgery. Most patients therefore are fully recovered within two years and continue to lead a full life without any side effects and without the threat of cancer.

The writer though has not been so fortunate. I have described him as "my most unlucky patient", the 'worst case scenario'. Following the operation he suffered all of the above problems to an alarming degree. This situation should occur in less than 1% of patients. Surgeons should be transparent about their outcomes so patients can be reassured that they are receiving high quality surgery. (An example of this can be found on the Birmingham Prostate Clinic website).

Despite this and having to undergo further treatment his determination and perseverance are such that he has handled the situation to a remarkable degree and continues to lead an active life with varied interests. His experiences are therefore not typical but provide a good example of how even the worst situation can be overcome with strength of character, faith and a sense of humour.

This book may benefit patients facing or undergoing treatment for prostate cancer.

Mr. Alan P. Doherty,
Consultant Urological Surgeon,
University Hospital of Birmingham.

INTRODUCTION

Being told that you have been diagnosed with cancer can be devastating, especially if you have followed a healthy lifestyle and are in good physical and mental health. The question "Why me?" comes to mind and could lead to negative thoughts of self-pity which in itself are harmful and can create a circle of despair. You may be concerned about the treatments offered, the possible side effects that may affect your lifestyle, the possible effect on your relationships as well as survival prospects. At this stage you must decide how you are going to face up to the challenges ahead. Time to take a positive and determined attitude!

In my case, tests for prostate cancer were initially indecisive with confirmation of the disease coming in the following year, this 'is it or is it not' period was a stressful experience in itself. When confirmation of the disease finally came I chose to take a positive approach, to 'fight it' and to continue to live life to the full. I had too much to live for to sit around moping! Following the diagnosis of prostate cancer I was sent to The Queen Elizabeth Hospital, Birmingham, where I was assessed and accepted for treatment and Urology Specialist Nurse Richard Gledhill was assigned to me. Specialist Nurses are highly trained and experienced and are among the unsung heroes of the N.H.S. providing advice, guidance and support to patients through often difficult and long-term treatment.

I was treated within four months of the diagnosis during which time I put myself through an intensive period of physical exercise to strengthen both body and mind for the ordeal ahead. This preparation culminated in a 'forced march' of around seventeen miles in seven hours with full pack following part of the British Front Line on the 1st of July 1916, the opening day of The Battle of The Somme, thus combining the exercise with one of my interests.

With the problems I experienced over the first few years after my treatment Richard became my rock, always there for me, always ready to help, at times a shoulder to cry on, a true friend. Most of our contact was by email and for some reason best known to himself he suggested, probably in jest, that I should write my life story. Having given it some thought I wrote what became the 'Prologue' to this work. With further encouragement from Richard I then set about writing this, my 'urological life story'.

If I have been the 'most unlucky patient' then the patient who became continent within three days of his operation and was starting to recover his sexual function in weeks must be the luckiest! (Michael Korda in his book 'Man to man. Surviving prostate cancer' gives an account of his experiences and had read a report of this case).

I hope that this account of my 'survival' will provide an inspiration to any man diagnosed with or being treated for prostate problems and an 'educational case study for the benefit of urologists worldwide'!

I apologise for any offence caused by the terms used (the majority of which can be found in the Oxford Dictionary from which most of the definitions are taken) or any embarrassment in reading it, and point out that it is in 'male humour' and in parts it contains 'slight' male exaggerations which should not be taken too seriously!

Most of this was written some three to five years after having the radical prostatectomy and succeeding operations, and with a few verses added later. In writing it I wish to thank the medical and support staff, and particularly the Specialist Nurses, who have helped and encouraged me through this, one of the most difficult periods in my life. Without their unstinting support, faith, a dogged determination to get through it, a loving wife and above all a wicked sense of humour, I might not have won. Many thanks also to Andy Watt for the cartoons, N.H. Cocks for helping with the script format, and Graham Fulford for accepting the work for publication.

It has been written in good faith for the benefit of others and is given to the Graham Fulford Charitable Trust to use in any way that may assist them in the good work they do in promoting awareness of prostate cancer.

George Sayell
2015

THE PROLOGUE[1]

In which I respond to Specialist Nurse Richard's request that I write my life story!

My dear Richard, I recall you did say,
    My life story I should write down one day,
Heed I have taken of your humble request,
    So by night and by day I am doing my best.

I will tell you the tale of my penis,
    A story of sadness and joy,
Of the trials the poor fellow has suffered,
    Since the days when I was but a boy.

I'll tell how he was a model of perfection,
    And how an operation put paid to all that,
How he became just a useless appendage,
    And my life became totally flat.

I'll tell of a nice nurse with injections,
    Men with white coats, probes and sharp knives,
And even a spell with a head-shrink,
    "My dear, Freud couldn't make that thing rise".

---

1   **prologue** *n.&v.* −n. **1a** a preliminary speech, poem etc., esp. introducing a play
(cf epilogue). **b** the actor speaking the prologue **2** *(usually followed by* to*).* any
act or event serving as an introduction. *Male urologists compare it to foreplay
before intercourse, although a recent survey found that 60% of married women
consider foreplay to be the main event and 35% have never experienced it − Ed.*

Oh, those dark days the poor fellow just dangled,
　　I felt like a eunuch, a failure, just grounded.
The treatments we tried, and all to no good,
　　Head hung low, distressed and confounded. [2]

And how the Yanks came to the rescue,
　　A vacuum pump that ended the pain,
And made my poor penis so happy,
　　To have his own way again.

I have my quill and I have my ink,
　　And my Concise Oxford is here by my side.
And so on parchment to you I'll tell all,
　　Rest assured, old chap, there is nothing I shall hide.

But, the problem you see, my brain is perverse,
　　And every thought has to come out in verse,
So be patient, please, my good friend,
　　For I will get there in the end........

2　**confounded** - *adj. colloq.* damned *(a confounded nuisance!).*

AN OVERVIEW OF MALE UROLOGY[3]

The human body is a very complex system, one of constant wonder and awe. In order to understand medical practice it is essential to have first a good grasp of the basic theory. This section provides a comprehensive and clear explanation of the physiology and psychology of male urology, far better than that found in any of the traditional medical textbooks! It is aimed primarily at the patient but it will also be to the benefit of the young Student Nurse and will enable the reader to appreciate fully the following case study.

This is a case study of urology,
　　And in particular that of the male,
I hope the things that I write about
　　Do not make the reader go pale.

Now I'd like to start with the penis,
　　A real little person no doubt,
With his own mind and sensitive feelings,
　　Not something to be just messed about.

He falls into the discipline of urology,
　　And is handled by professionals worldwide,[4]
And the ability to keep him working,
　　Is what sets these people aside.

A man is very sensitive about his penis,
　　Best not to comment on its size,
Unless you tell him he's got a whopper,
　　And bring a tear of joy to his eyes.

3　**urology** *n.* the scientific study of the urinary system.
　　urologic *adj.* **urologist** *n.*
4　*In this context by medical professionals – Ed.*

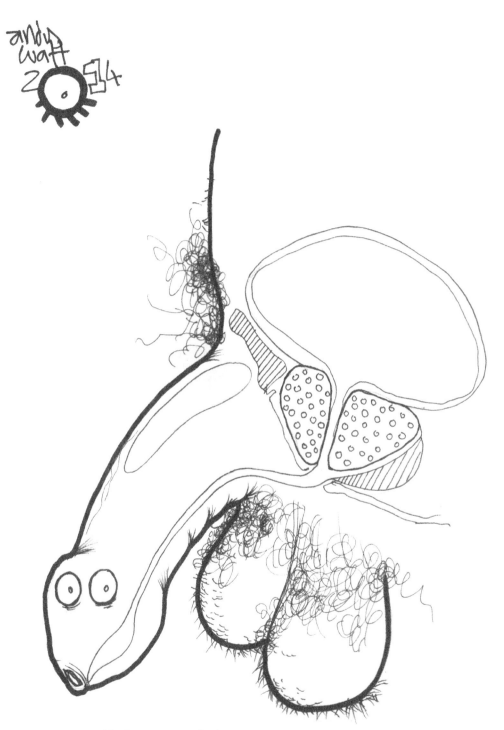

'a real little person no doubt'

In animal anatomy he is unique,
	A point on which I really must dwell,
For at the sight of an attractive female
	You should see the little chap swell.

For this we thank the corpus cavernosa,
	Erectile tubes within the man's dick, [5]
On command they are pumped up with blood, [6]
	And the penis becomes as stiff as a stick.

Now when this physical change happens,
	And as part of nature's great plan,
The brain migrates to the penis,
	And controls the mind of the man.

And when he is in this condition,
	With your last shirt you can place any bets
That the man will have no inhibitions,
	For a stiff penis does not have regrets. [7]

This is of course part of his function,
	As he grows up to six times his size,
But as part of the male psychology,
	If this fails the man mentally dies.

Now the penis is a man's pride and joy,
	But urology involves other parts too.
He's part of a complex system,
	Which I'll now explain to you.

At the top of the tree is the bladder,
	The urine is stored in this sac,
In the young man it's the size of a kitbag
	But like an eggcup in the elderly chap.

---

5   **dick.** n. 1 Brit. colloq. (in certain set phrases) fellow; person (clever dick).
    2 *coarse sl.* the penis.
6   *It is said that a man's erection starts in the brain which sends a message to the
    penis ordering it to 'Action Stations'. - Ed.*
7   *A common expression in the 1950s, drummed into every young lady by her
    mother, was 'a standing penis has no conscience'. - Ed.*

My story will mention the prostate,
    A small gland twixt bladder and dick.
It mixes the seminal cocktail, [8]
    That makes the poor penis be sick.

Now the tube to the penis is the urethra,
    Through which urine and semen doth flow,
A delicate tube so easily damaged,
    As my case study will certainly show.

Now the sphincter is nothing to do with the Sphinx.
    It's a muscular ring by the prostate
To stop you wetting your pants between wees [9]
    By closing the urethra like a flood gate.

Now another essential is the testicle,
    Of these most men will have two [10]
So young boys can play pocket billiards,
    They're possibly known as the 'balls' by you.

But the testicles have a secondary function,
    The production of litres of semen,
Minute tadpole like potholing creatures,
    Whose sole intent is to fertilise women.

Now the testicles hang in a large pouch
    The medical term for which is the scrotum. [11]
It keeps the testicles safe and cool,
    And dangles between penis and rectum.

---

8   **seminal** *adj.* 1 of or relating to seed, semen or reproduction.
    2 germinal. 3 rudimentary, undeveloped. 4 (of ideas etc.) providing the basis for
    future development.

9   **wee** *n.* esp. *Brit.sl.* = WEE-WEE. **wee-wee** *n.&v.* esp. *Brit. sl. —n.*
    1 the act or an instance of urinating. 2 urine *—v.intr.*

10   *There have been exceptions, as quoted in the Colonel Bogey marching song,*
    "Hitler has only got one ball". - Ed

11   **scrotum** *n.* (*pl* **scrota** or **scrotums**) a pouch of skin containing the testicles.
    It is reputed that in the old 'Wild West' the scrotums of slain Indians made
    excellent souvenir tobacco pouches. - Ed.

The vas deferens connect the testicles to the prostate,
    Tubes with a name that sounds Dutch.
The sperm is pumped up through these pipes,
    Beyond that I can't add very much.

If we now put the whole lot together
    We have 'The male urology kit'.
And by working together in harmony,
    Each and every part does its bit.

So that dear reader is male urology,
    Which you now understand so much better,
But there's a related item I really must mention,
    It is of course, the ubiquitous 'French Letter'! [12]

They come in various shapes, colours and sizes,
    And are made of the finest latex,
There are many makers and brand names worldwide,
    But the finest of all is the British 'Durex'.

They're now rolled on the phallus by the liberated young lady, [13]
    Anxious to avoid pregnancy, Aids and a dose of the Pox.
And the young man should not be embarrassed,
    It's no different to having her pull up your socks!

I can now tell you the tale of my penis,
    A story of both sadness and joy,
Of the trials the little chap has suffered
    Since the days when I was but a boy.

---

12 **condom** *n.* a rubber sheath worn on the penis during sexual intercourse as a
    contraceptive or to prevent infection. *It is thought that these ubiquitous items*
    are so named having been invented by a Colonel Condon in the 17th Century to
    protect his soldiers from the 'French disease'. - Ed.
13 **phallus**. *n.* (*pl.* **phalli** or **phalluses**) 1 the (esp. erect) penis.
    2 an image of this as a symbol of generative power in nature.

MY EARLY YEARS.

Those halcyon days of youth we all yearn back to, when the sun shone all summer and we had not a care in the world.

Once upon a time I was just a little tyke,
    A little boy so meek and mild,
Who thought willies were only for peeing; [14]
    Yes, I was such an innocent sweet child.

To a boy urology means nothing,
    Football and school were my all,
I'd happily spend all day with my books,
    Or out on the pitch with a ball.

And then I became a youth,
    And my body began to grow,
Whiskers on my face and elsewhere,
    But the biggest change was down below.

And as I became a young man
    My interests began to change
I started to look at the girls
    And they no longer seemed so strange.

---

14   **willy** *n.* (also **willie**) (*pl.* –**ies**) *Brit. sl.* the penis.
pee *v.* & *n. colloq.* –*v.* (**pees**, **peed**) 1 *intr.* urinate. 2 *tr.* pass (urine, blood etc.) from the bladder.

Oh, I then was so proud of 'Little William',
    With his 'Dr.Jekyll and Mr.Hyde trick, [15]
And as he became 'Big Bad Willy',
    I had a really magnificent dick.

He was of a size unimaginable,
    To the girls a most awesome sight,
For many a maiden first spotted him,
    And immediately fainted with fright.

And he could also wee like a carthorse,
    With a range of five metres at least,
And pee upwards two metres or more,
    An Olympic champ of a beast!

Now for years I spent my nights courting,
    And broke many a young ladies heart,
But mine was oft broken as well,
    For it's always so hard to part.

I decided to settle down in my twenties,
    And needed to look for a wife.
At a teachers' ball I met a young lady,
    The most wonderful thing in my life.

15 *In "The Strange Case of Dr.Jekyll and Mr.Hyde", R.L.Stevenson tells the story of how the virtuous Dr. Jekyll took mind-changing drugs and became the evil Mr.Hyde. I have often wondered if it was this natural phenomenon that was the inspiration for the novel. - Ed.*

I courted her for less than a year,
    For this lady and I were soon wed
And my penis had the time of his life,
    Doing his duty in the marital bed.

And in time he sired our two daughters,
    Oh what sweet lovely children were they.
Unfortunately they turned into teenagers,
    And that's when I began to go grey.

In those days I was so fit and healthy,
    Cycling, walking, archery and more,
With hobbies that kept the mind busy,
    And illness never crossed my front door.

But I was just a typical young man,
    With no idea of the future in store,
How these halcyon days would be over,
    And he would function like this no more.

Oh, the joys of once being so young,
    Oh why couldn't the clock have stood still?
Oh why did I have to grow old,
    And sooner or later fall ill?

DISASTER STRIKES

*At 67 I was extremely fit and active for a man of my age, and living a full
life. My wife and I were enjoying good sex and were totally unprepared for the
life changing events that were about to unfold.*

Now every year the doc did a blood check,
    Including a test called the P.S.A., [16]
And the result each year was "you're fine",
    Despite me peeing every hour of the day. [17]

Now the GFCT does these tests also, [18]
    And their sessions had a talk by a doc,
So I went along and gave them a sample,
    And the result was a bit of a shock.

For the result was an 'amber warning', [19]
    Did I have cancer or was I quite clear?
So a month later we repeated the test
    And this result was not what I wanted to hear.

So the doc sent me off for a biopsy, [20]
    A large probe shoved up my rectum,
Twelve painful jabs in the prostate
    And I went home with a very sore bum.

---

16 *Prostate Specific Antogen. A protein in the blood, manufactured by
the prostate. The level of PSA in the blood may indicate problems in the
prostate. – Ed.*
17 *Urinating frequently can be a symptom of prostate problems. - Ed.*
18 GFCT. The 'Graham Fulford Charitable Trust.' *Ed.*
19 *The Trust sends each patient a report giving the actual PSA value and
a 'Red, Amber or Green' indication of severity taking into account the
patient's age. - Ed.*
20 **biopsy.** *n.* (*pl.* **–ies**) the examination of tissues removed from a living
body to discover the presence, cause, or extent of a disease.

But the biopsy was indefinite also,
    Suspicious cells but not the disease,
Which left me in a state of limbo,
    Full of fear, trepidation and unease.

So I kept taking the PSA test,
    Anxious that every result would be low
And it went up and down for a while,
    Then one day the result was rather a blow.

And so I was sent back to the hospital,
    Once again to bare my backside,
Held down by two big nurses,
    And twelve more jabs right up the inside.

And this time I was struck down with shock,
    For cancer in me had been found,
It felt like the end of the world,
    And I collapsed in tears on the ground.

Then a very nice nurse picked me up,
    And comforted me in her most caring way,
And told me it was not the end,
    And I would live on for many a day.

The cancer was still in the prostate,
    And was found at the earliest stage,
None of it had escaped so far
    And I could still live to a decent old age.

And so promptly to the Q.E. I was sent, [21]
    Where the consultant and I discussed what to do.
I was interviewed and counselled for hours
    On operations, radiotherapy and hormones too.

---

21   *The Queen Elizabeth Hospital, Birmingham. Ed.*

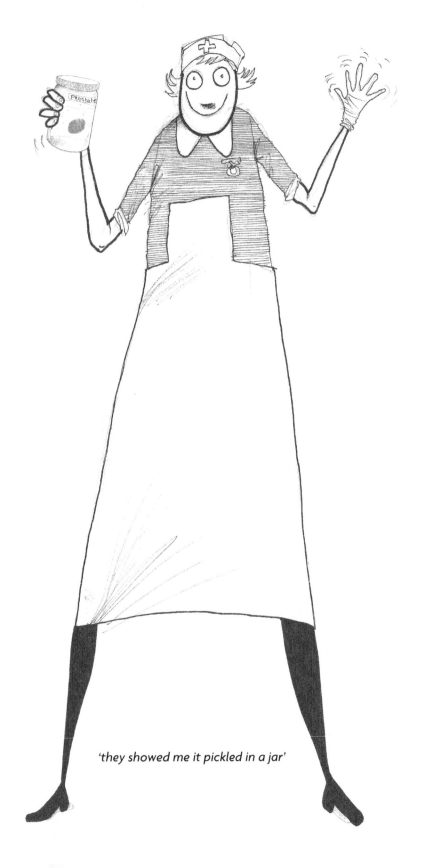

'they showed me it pickled in a jar'

We soon decided I should go in for an op, [22]
    Take the damn thing out and be done,
This as an engineer I could understand,
    Psychologically, the only option.

And at this time I met Nurse Richard,
    Who in no time did put me right,
That I wouldn't be discharged the next day,
    For I'd be starting a very hard fight.

So in due course I went back there,
    To spend the longest night of my life!
Lying in the ward wondering what the future would be
    After meeting a man with a very sharp knife.

And out it came the next morning,
    They showed me it pickled in a jar, [23]
Awaiting slicing and inspection in the lab,
    To see if the cancer had yet spread afar.

In time I went home from hospital,
    And spent many a week in pain,
Starting my long recovery,
    To become a fit man again.

But that was not the end of the story,
    Not time for a joyful shout.
For what I hadn't bargained for was,
    I was left a bit 'buggered about'. [24]

---

22 **op** *n. colloq.* operation (in surgical and military senses). *In this case to remove the prostate by keyhole surgery (Laparoscopic Radical Prostatectomy) – Ed.*
23 *On coming round from the anaesthetic I asked the Theatre Nurse to show it to me. Not many men can say they've seen their prostate! – Ed.*
24 **bugger** *n., v. & int. coarse sl.* (except in sense 2 of n. and 3 of v.) Usually considered a taboo word. **–n. 1** an unpleasant or awkward person or thing (*the bugger won't fit*). **2** a person who commits buggery. *–v.tr.* **1** as an exclamation of annoyance (bugger the thing!) **2** (often followed by *up*) Brit. **a** ruin; spoil (*really buggered it up; no good, it's buggered*). **bugger about** (or **around**) (often foll. by *with*) **1** mess about. **2** mislead; persecute. **bugger-all** nothing. **bugger off** (often in *imper.*) go away.

ONGOING PROBLEMS

Having the prostate removed was just the start of the problems. I had expected with my level of fitness to make a quick and full recovery. Incontinence at this stage is normal but little did I realize what else I was about to face.

For week after week I suffered,
    With abdomen and penis in pain.
Would there be no end to this,
    Would I ever be the same again?

And then one night disaster did strike,
    The poor little chap couldn't pee,
Just drip, drip, drip in the toilet,
    And this certainly worried me. [25]

Now the reason for this was puzzling,
    Until Nurse Richard explained it to me,
The catheter had damaged the urethra, [26]
    And the scarring was stopping the wee.

---

25 *This was a very frightening situation, realizing that it could lead to a medical emergency. That this was a rare post-op problem was no consolation when regularly spending time during the cold night trying to dribble into the toilet and not down my legs, while almost asleep! – Ed.*
26 **catheter** *n. Med.* a tube for insertion into a body cavity for introducing or removing fluid. *In this case urine from the bladder to an external bag during recovery after the operation. Following my experience the hospital changed the specification of catheter to prevent further such problems - Ed.*

So it was back to the QE again,
    "Optical Urethrotomy is our trade." [27]
There they cut the inside of my poor penis,
    But not a 'drip' of difference it made.

So a few months later I had to go back
    And they cut the poor fellow again,
With no hope of doing any good,
    In return for suffering the pain.

So I was then sent to 'Russells Hall',
    A large hospital in Dudley town,
Where a surgeon does fantastic work,
    A man of TV fame and renown.

He is a specialist in urethroplasty, [28]
    A solution I had to embrace,
He made me a brand new urethra,
    Now I pee through the side of my face!

---

27 *An operation whereby an instrument is passed through the penis and up into the urethra and a small slit made in the restricted part of the urethra to widen it. - Ed.*
28 *The replacement of a damaged part of the urethra with skin taken from elsewhere in the body, in my case from the inside of the mouth. - Ed.*

FAILURE TO STAND UP FOR ONE'S RIGHTS

Although the urethral problem had been fixed that was not the end of my problems. I had been doing exercises to strengthen the muscles around the sphincter to eliminate urine leakage and as advised had put sex 'on the back burner' for 12 months.

Poor William still knackered was he,
　　A complete urological wreck,
In my pants he did nothing but pee
　　And all day just gazed down at the deck.

And then one night at bedtime,
　　An earth-shattering shock I had,
For despite the romantic setting,
　　Little William just curled up, oh so sad.

So a little blue tablet the doc to me gave, [29]
　　"Take one at night, it will do the trick",
But the little chap, still lifeless was he,
　　And I was just an impotent prick. [30]

---

29 *Tablets containing sildenafil intended to increase blood flow into the penis to produce an erection. One of a number of excellent treatments for Erectile Dysfunction (impotence) but ineffective if the nerves connecting the brain to the penis have been cut during removal of the prostate. - Ed.*
30 **prick** *v. & n. –v.* **1** *tr.* pierce slightly; make a small hole in. **2** *tr.* (foll by *off, out*) mark (*esp.* a pattern) with small holes or dots. **3** *tr.* trouble mentally (*my conscience is pricking me*). **4** *intr.* feel a pricking sensation. **5** *intr.* (foll. by *at, intro* etc.) make a thrust as if to prick. **6** *coarse sl.* **a** the penis. **b** *derog.* (as a term of contempt) a person. Usually considered a taboo usage. *Typical usage – 'you useless prick'. - A pun! The use of 'prick' as a noun may be related to its use as a verb and the similarity between 'to prick' and 'to penetrate'. Hence the graffiti seen in a play area "Virginity is like a balloon, one prick and it's gone"- Ed.*

So the next thing they tried was a pellet, [31]
 "This will give you the desired reaction.
Just insert it in the end of the penis,
 And in five minutes you'll have an erection".

Now the first time I tried with one pellet,
 And gave him a good massage as well,
But the little chap hardly woke up
 And no sign of him starting to swell.

So I tried again with two pellets,
 Inserting them as far in as I could,
Waited for at least five minutes,
 But still they did me no good.

Then came a nice nurse with a hypo, [32]
 And smiling injected him with glee,
"How bizarre!" she cried, [33]
 As he still drooped by her side,
And then, on the floor, did a wee!

Bizarre to me it certainly was not,
 So desperate was I for the horn, [34]
To suffer the needle in my dick for nowt,
 Sent me home all shattered and forlorn.

---

31 *Small suppositories containing Prostaglandin (Alprostadil) are inserted into the urethra where they melt into and are absorbed by the surrounding area. The chemical causes an increase in the blood flow in the corpus cavernosa to produce an erection. - Ed.*
32 *A hypodermic containing Prostaglandin (Alprostadil) which is injected into the penis. The chemical causes an increase in the blood flow in the corpus cavernosa to produce an erection. – Ed.*
33 **bizarre** *adj.* strange in appearance or effect; eccentric; grotesque.
34 **horn.** *n* & *v.* –*n.* **1 a** a hard permanent outgrowth, often curved and pointed, on hoofed mammals, found singly, in pairs, or one in front of another. **b** the structure of a horn, consisting of a core of bone encased in keratinized skin. **2** anything resembling or compared to a horn in shape.

But the nice nurse tried many more times,
    With doses of increasing strength
And I plucked up the courage to try too,
    But he grew not a micron in length. [35]

But now the poor chap was like a pin cushion,
    And Peyronie was my greatest dread, [36]
So every night I checked with a straight-edge,
    The last thing before going to bed.

They then gave to me a nice pump, [37]
    An American invention no doubt,
But despite being a clever old boy,
    I just couldn't quite fathom it out.

So the poor chap just hung limp and floppy,
    Oh dear, what on earth was I to do?
This was no way for a man to be,
    Just think, what if it happened to you?

---

35 **micron** n. one millionth of a metre. *The metric equivalent of the British engineer's 'flea's dick', the term commonly used with Imperial measurements. - Ed.*
36 *Peyronie's disease. A connective tissue disorder causing pain, abnormal curvature, erectile dysfunction, loss of girth and shortening.*
Example:
    There was a young man from Kent,
    Whose tool was decidedly bent.
    To save so much trouble,
    He shoved it up double,
    And instead of coming * *he went! - Ed.*

* come v. sl. Have a sexual orgasm. n. sl. Semen ejaculated at a sexual orgasm
37 *A penile vacuum pump. A device comprising a hollow tube into which the limp penis is placed and with a vacuum pump at the other end. Blood is drawn into the penis creating an erection and the erection maintained by fitting a rubber ring around the base of the penis. - Ed.*

PSYCHOSEXUAL THERAPY

In the majority of cases 'erectile dysfunction' is readily cured by the use of oral tablets or one of the Alprostadil methods, or the patient readily takes to the Vacuum Pump.
In my case all of these treatments had been unsuccessful despite all the efforts of the 'nice nurse'.
It was time to take a different approach. My last chance!

And then the nice nurse, an idea she had,
 "The problem is your brain, not the spout,
To the hospital headshrinker I'll send you, [38]
 I'm sure she can sort you right out."

For months it had been failure after failure,
 And each time I became more forlorn.
"Performance anxiety is the root of your problem! [39]
 Therapy will get you back on top form."

And so off I went to the shrink,
 And we talked through all of my life.
I spent many an hour with her,
 And they had a session as well with my wife.

We talked about my life in general,
 I told of the good times and also the bad,
My sex life, our marriage and my problems,
 And each session left me feeling so sad.

---

38 **headshrinker** *sl.* a psychiatrist.
39 *Performance anxiety. Inability to relax through anticipation of failure causes the body to release chemicals which will counter the effects of the medication. - Ed.*

And in time the headshrinker assessed me,
    And it's difficult to tell it in verse,
"No-hoper" said she, "as you are, you will be",
    And I just couldn't have felt any worse!

"It's no good my dear fellow,
    Your days of sex are now gone,
You're only torturing yourself.
    Stop trying - you must learn to move on!

The best I can do for you dear patient,
    For penetration is just beyond hope,
Is to teach you to live without sex,
    And the two of you will learn how to cope.

You can express your love in other ways,
    And you'll be no less of a man for that."
But for me this felt like a death sentence,
    A eunuch, less use than a poor old prat.[40]

I felt like a neutered tomcat,
    When approached by a queen on heat,
And tries his best to mount her
    But then has to admit defeat. [41]

But the headshrinker was very professional,
    For the problem I now understood,
But for me to give up would be failure,
    I just had to do all that I possibly could.

The nice nurse sadly to me had to say,
    "I can do no more; we've tried every known fix".
Now this was not what I wanted to hear,
    It flattened me like a ton of house bricks.

---

40 **prat** n. sl. 1 Brit. a silly or foolish person. 2 the buttocks.
41 This was an actual occurrence. We had two such cats, both Siamese, the end result being the male retreated looking absolutely dejected whilst being attacked by the furious and sexually frustrated female. - Ed.

DESPERATION AND THE SOLUTION

For months following the psychosexual therapy I was in a state of 'depression'. To be incapable of having sex made me feel less than a real man. I could see that the need was as much psychological as physical. The 'nice nurse', despite all her help and enthusiasm, could do no more for me and I was now on my own.

Oh, those dark days the poor penis just dangled,
 I felt like a eunuch, a failure, just grounded.
The treatments we'd tried, and all to no good,
 Head hung low, distressed and confounded.

So, on the web a solution I did seek,
 These new implants looked just like a winner, [42]
But put off was I at the thought of the knife,
 And a pump in the scrotum, what a killer!

So out came my trusty old pump,
 And I practiced by night and by day,
Big Bad Willy so desperate was he,
 To stand up and get his own way.

---

42 *Flexible Penile implants. Inflatable tubes in the shaft of the penis operated by a pump in the scrotum to enable an erection capable of penetration. - Ed.*

At last when I found I could manage it,
  Eight inches was there in my hand!
A tool to satisfy any woman!
  'Oh boy, by George, what a stand!'

This pump is a fantastic contraption,
  The inventor is certainly no fool,
For in goes a teeny-weeny penis,
  And out comes a whopping great tool!

So if my pride and joy is my penis,
  My sanity has been saved by my pump,
For in the days when my penis was useless,
  The pump got me over the hump! [43]

I may not need to have sex very often,
  It's just knowing I can do it that matters.
A man should not put up with E.D.
  And feel that his life is in tatters.

---

43 **hump** *n. & v. —n.* **1** a rounded protuberance on the back of a camel etc., or as an abnormality on a person's back. **2** a rounded raised mass of earth etc. **3** *course sl.* have sexual intercourse with. In sense 3 usually considered a taboo word.

'at last when I found I could manage it'

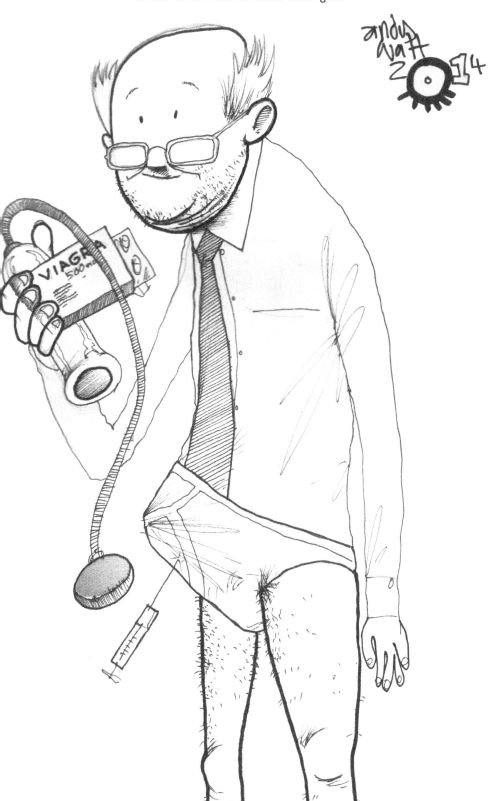

A PENSIONER IN NAPPIES

Having found a solution to the impotence problem I felt more of a man again,
but I was still left with the problem of constant leakage. This varied according to
the level of activity and was controlled by the use of pads.

But I still have the problem of leakage,
    Just drip, drip, drip in a pad, [44]
This goes on twenty-four seven,
    And at times it makes me feel oh so sad.

I leak when I cough, I leak when I sneeze,
    And I can't enjoy a good fart. [45]
For to squeeze the muscles whilst breaking wind [46]
    Is an almost impossible art.

Wearing pads is a bit of a bugbear, [47]
    I get through a dozen a week,
And I never walk past a urinal
    For the more you piddle, the less you will leak! [48]

But then you can have another op,
    A sling fitted under the bladder,
It relieves the pressure on the sphincter,
    And reduces the chance of disaster.

---

44 *continence pads worn inside underpants. - Ed.*
45 **fart** *v. & n. coarse sl. −v.intr.* 1 emit wind from the anus. 2 (foll. by *about, around*) behave foolishly: waste time. − *n.* 1 an emission of wind from the anus. 2 an unpleasant person. Usually considered a taboo word.
A natural bodily function, the cause of great mirth and a competitive sport in many offices. From the Middle English 'ferten', 'to break wind'. Ed.
46 *Post radical prostatectomy patients are taught pelvic floor muscle strengthening exercises to reduce leakage. − Ed.*
47 **bugbear**. *n.* 1 a cause of annoyance or anger; a *bête-noire*. 2 an object of baseless fear. 3 *archaic* a sort of hobgoblin or any being invoked to intimidate children.
48 **piddle** *v. & n. colloq. − v.intr.* 1 *colloq.* urinate (used esp. by or to children). 2 work or act in a trifling way. 3 (as **piddling** *adj.) colloq.* trivial; trifling. *n. colloq.*

Or they might offer you a new sphincter,
    A thing designed by a medical geek,
With pipe work and controls in the scrotum
    Controlling a clamp that prevents any leak.

But these would mean going back to the QE,
    Being cut open again with the knife,
With complications and additional risks also,
    But I've had enough of that stuff for one life!

They've offered me the 'piddle-tube' option, [49]
    It goes from willy to a bag on the calf,
It's certainly an alternative solution,
    But it strikes me as a bit of a laugh.

But it does have one advantage,
    If the bag is full when walking in town, [50]
Just kneel down *'to do up your shoe lace'*,
    Open the tap, and drain the bag down!

And then there is the penile clamp,
    A bulldog clip that will stop any leak,
Just unclip it to go for a wee, [51]
    But the poor chap would look quite a freak.

And so I am left incontinent,
    The Cross I will always have to bear,
Unpleasant but not life threatening,
    And preferable to the big C down there.

---

49 *A penile sheath connected by a tube to a drainable collection bag on the leg. - Ed.*
50 *I had an unfortunate experience testing one of these – I was having a good wee into the bag when the sheath slipped of the penis causing me to pee in my trousers and fill my boots. Fortunately I wasn't in town at the time! - Ed.*
51 *These devices can only be worn for a limited time when they must be temporarily removed to restore blood flow to the end of the penis, not always convenient. - Ed.*

SUMMARY

In which I give good advice and encouragement to the patient and remind the doctors and nurses of the importance of looking at the patient as a whole person.

To the chap diagnosed with prostate big C,
    I'm afraid the treatment is a bit of a pain,
But don't despair or lose hope old fellow,
    For in time you'll be your old self again.

Do get plenty of exercise and fresh air,
    Maintain a healthy mental and physical state.
Golf, squash, running or walking are all fine,
    But for me, cycling and gliding are great.

Find time for your hobbies as well,
    Whatever you used to enjoy,
Take your mind off the problems for a while,
    Go back to doing what you did as a boy.

Have faith, courage, and strength,
    Don't listen to what the pessimists say,
For you can battle your way through it,
    Yes, you can beat it, just take it day by day.

Most patients don't suffer from problems,
    Their bodies recover quite soon,
They hardly ever pee in their pants
    And their willies still gaze up at the moon.

At times you may feel despondent,
    And your problems will make you feel down,
But keep laughing at the situation,
    Wipe from your face that terrible frown.

Tell your nurse all about your problems,
      Spill out your tales of woe,
For they are there to help you
      And to see your confidence grow.

Just remember you'll win your way through it,
      There's someone less lucky than you,
Dementia, paraplegics, blindness and worse,
      M.S., renal failure and Parkinson's too!

I know because I've been there,
      I've had my difficult times,
I've laughed at the state of my willy,
      As I'm telling you in these rhymes.

Now I've been the most unlucky patient,
      Your case will be easier than mine,
And if I can battle my way through it,
      I'm sure that you'll soon be fine.

And despite all the problems I've had,
      The thing that has made it worthwhile,
My P.S.A. is almost zero,
      AND THAT'S WHY I'VE GOT A GREAT SMILE!

And if you feel like not having the treatment,
      The thought of impotence is your worst dread,
Have a good think about the bigger picture,
      For you'll get no erection if you're dead!

For if your member becomes useless, [52]
    Tablets should enable you to cope,
Or he'll stiffen up with Alprostadil,
    And even if that fails there's still hope.

So then dear fellow, keep a grin on your face,
    Get a pump and use it at night,
Ten minutes pumping and thirty minutes humping, [53]
    Your sex life will again be alright.

And as for the young man that mocks you,
    Considers your pump the most hilarious sight,
Now that fool 'comes his lot' in thirty seconds, [54]
    While you can keep at it all night! [55]

And if you find when he's limp and floppy,
    'Spanking the monkey' is difficult to do, [56]
Get yourself a ladies' vibrator,
    And see what it can do for you!

52 **member** *n.* **1** a person belonging to a society, team etc. **2** (**Member**) a person formally elected to take part in the proceedings of certain organisations. **3** (also *attrib.*) a part or branch of a political body **4** a constituent portion of a complex structure. **5** a part of a sentence, equation, group of figures, mathematical set, etc. **6 a** any part or organ of the body, esp. a limb. **b** = PENIS.
53 **hump** *(See previous. Ed.)*
54 *To 'come one's lot' is to ejaculate. I first heard this expression in the factory around 1960 when a man shouted loudly to a young office girl who was going out with his apprentice "Is he no good to you K...., does he come his lot too quick?". This offensive behaviour was considered acceptable in those days.*
55 *The constriction rings used to maintain the erection can be kept in place for about 30 minutes which for most people should be sufficient for sex. They then have to be removed to enable blood circulation through the penis but after a short period the process can be repeated, and repeated, and .... - Ed.*
56 *'Spanking the monkey'. One of many slang terms for masturbation. - Ed.*

And to all urologists I really must say,
    However bright you think you may be,
Don't forget that a chap's little penis,
    Is there to do more than just pee.

Urology is not just medical science,
    Operations that are great fun to perform.
It's about the sex problems of real people,
    Creating a physical and emotional storm.

And now I'm a real man again,
    My story has come to its end,
And I'm sure you can tell, dear reader,
    Why my nurse is my very best friend!

'Never give up, never ever.'
'Laugh and the world laughs with you, cry and you cry alone'.

POSTSCRIPT (FEBRUARY 2015)

Seven years after the Radical Prostatectomy and subsequent operations it is time to take stock of the changes that have taken place since.

The highest measured PSA reading since the Radical Prostatectomy is 0.02, before treatment it was 6.7.

Internal inspections have shown that the 'new' urethra is sound and that the condition of the sphincter has gradually improved. As a result urine flow rates are good and over the years there has been a reduction in urine leakage.

Whereas the penile injections were ineffective when originally tried, a recent trial 'showed promise' and with an increased sensitivity in the glans (head of penis).

Time is a great healer!

REFERENCES

Definitions taken from Fowler H.W., F.G.Fowler and R.E.Allen (eds.) *The Concise Oxford Dictionary of Current English* (Eighth Edition) (Oxford: Clarendon, 1990)

Michael Korda. MAN TO MAN. SURVIVING PROSTATE CANCER. (Little Brown and Company, 1997. Previously published in the United States)

Lightning Source UK Ltd.
Milton Keynes UK
UKOW06f2114070915

258217UK00002B/49/P